AVERY WRIGHT

The Ultimate Guide to Meal Planning

Contents

Thank You

Thank you for reading The Ultimate Guide to Meal Planning. We hope that this guide has provided you with valuable information and strategies to make meal planning a successful and enjoyable part of your routine. By planning healthy, budget-friendly meals that can be prepared in advance, you can save time, reduce stress, and take control of your health and budget. Remember to stay organized, stay flexible, and have fun with the process. Happy meal planning!

Avery Wright

1

Introduction

Meal planning is the process of organizing and preparing meals ahead of time. This involves selecting recipes, shopping for ingredients, and preparing meals in advance. Meal planning has become increasingly popular in recent years due to its numerous benefits. In this chapter, we will discuss the importance of meal planning and the benefits it can bring to your life.

The Importance of Meal Planning

Meal planning is important for several reasons. First and foremost, it can save you time. By planning your meals ahead of time, you can avoid last-minute trips to the grocery store and time spent figuring out what to cook. This can free up time in your day for other activities, such as spending time with family, exercising, or pursuing a hobby.

Meal planning can also save you money. When you plan your meals ahead of time, you can make a shopping list and stick to it, which can help you avoid impulse purchases and unnecessary spending. You can also take advantage of sales and coupons to save even more money.

Meal planning can also help you eat healthier. When you plan your meals ahead of time, you have more control over what you eat. You can select recipes that are nutrient-dense and well-balanced, and avoid relying on convenience foods that are often high in calories, sugar, and unhealthy fats.

Finally, meal planning can help reduce food waste. When you plan your meals ahead of time, you can buy only what you need and use up ingredients before they go bad. This can help you save money and reduce your environmental footprint.

Benefits of Meal Planning

The benefits of meal planning are numerous and can positively impact your health, finances, and overall wellbeing. Here are some of the key benefits:

Saves time: By planning your meals ahead of time, you can avoid last-minute trips to the grocery store and time spent figuring out what to cook.

Saves money: Meal planning can help you stick to a budget and avoid impulse purchases, which can save you money in the long run.

Improves nutrition: Meal planning allows you to choose

healthy, nutrient-dense foods and avoid relying on convenience foods that are often high in calories, sugar, and unhealthy fats.

Reduces food waste: By planning your meals ahead of time, you can buy only what you need and use up ingredients before they go bad, reducing food waste and saving money.

Promotes variety: Meal planning encourages you to try new recipes and experiment with different ingredients, which can help you discover new favorite foods and prevent boredom.

Reduces stress: By planning your meals ahead of time, you can reduce the stress of mealtime decision-making and ensure that you always have a healthy, satisfying meal on hand.

Supports weight loss: By choosing healthy, nutrient-dense foods and avoiding high-calorie convenience foods, meal planning can support weight loss and weight management.

Encourages family time: Meal planning can be a fun and collaborative activity that involves the whole family, encouraging quality time spent together.

In summary, meal planning is an important and beneficial habit to cultivate. It can save you time and money, improve your nutrition, reduce food waste, promote variety, reduce stress, support weight loss, and encourage family time. In the next sections of this guide, we will explore the strategies and tips for effective meal planning to help you achieve these benefits.

2

Setting Goals

Meal planning is a process that involves setting goals and priorities in order to make informed decisions about what to eat. When it comes to setting goals for meal planning, there are three key areas to consider: dietary needs, budget limits, and time constraints.

Determining Dietary Needs

The first step in setting goals for meal planning is to determine your dietary needs. This includes considering your personal health goals, any dietary restrictions or allergies, and any cultural or ethical food preferences. For example, if you are trying to lose weight, you may want to focus on recipes that are lower in calories and higher in protein. If you have a food allergy or intolerance, you will need to avoid certain ingredients. If you follow a vegan or vegetarian diet, you will need to plan meals that are free of animal products.

To determine your dietary needs, it can be helpful to consult with a healthcare professional, such as a registered dietitian, who can provide personalized recommendations based on your health history and goals.

Setting Budget Limits

The second step in setting goals for meal planning is to consider your budget limits. This includes determining how much you can afford to spend on groceries each week or month, as well as identifying strategies for saving money, such as buying in bulk, using coupons, or shopping at discount stores.

When setting a budget for meal planning, it can be helpful to track your spending for a few weeks to get a sense of how much you typically spend on groceries. You can then set a target budget that is realistic and achievable, while still allowing you to buy nutritious and satisfying foods.

Considering Time Constraints

The third step in setting goals for meal planning is to consider your time constraints. This includes determining how much time you have available to prepare meals each day or week, as well as identifying strategies for saving time, such as batch cooking or using a slow cooker.

When considering your time constraints, it can be helpful to think about your schedule for the week ahead and identify any days when you will have more or less time for meal preparation. You can then plan your meals accordingly, selecting recipes that are quick and easy to prepare on busy days, and more elaborate recipes for days when you have more time.

In addition to these three key areas, it can also be helpful to set goals for meal planning in other areas, such as taste preferences, environmental impact, or cultural traditions. By setting clear goals in these areas, you can ensure that your meal planning efforts are aligned with your values and priorities.

Tips for Achieving Your Goals

Once you have set your goals for meal planning, there are several tips and strategies that can help you achieve them.

Use a meal planning template: A meal planning template can help you stay organized and ensure that you are meeting your dietary needs and budget limits. You can create your own template or use one of the many free templates available online.

Plan for leftovers: When planning your meals, consider making extra servings that you can eat for lunch or dinner the next day. This can save you time and money, while also ensuring that you have healthy, satisfying meals on hand.

Use seasonal produce: Buying produce that is in season can be a cost-effective way to add variety to your meals. Seasonal produce is often fresher and more flavorful than out-of-season produce, and it is typically less expensive.

Batch cook: Batch cooking involves preparing a large batch of a recipe, such as chili or soup, and freezing portions for later use. This can be a time-saving strategy that allows you to have healthy meals on hand when you are short on time.

Shop at discount stores: Shopping at discount stores, such as Aldi or Lidl, can be a cost-effective way to buy groceries. These stores often offer quality products at a lower cost than traditional grocery stores, allowing you to save money while still getting the ingredients you need for your meal planning.

Utilize your pantry: Keep your pantry stocked with healthy, shelf-stable items, such as canned goods, grains, and spices. This can help you create meals quickly and easily, without having to run to the store for ingredients.

Be flexible: Remember that meal planning is not set in stone. Be willing to adjust your plan if necessary, and allow for some spontaneity and flexibility in your meals.

Track your progress: Keeping track of your progress can help you stay motivated and see the positive changes that meal planning can bring to your health and budget. Consider using a food journal or app to track your meals, grocery expenses, and progress towards your goals.

Reward yourself: Finally, remember to reward yourself for your hard work and progress. This can help you stay motivated and make meal planning a habit. Treat yourself to a night out, a small gift, or a special meal to celebrate your successes.

By following these tips and strategies, you can achieve your goals for meal planning and enjoy the benefits of healthy, budget-friendly meals that can be prepared in advance. Remember to stay organized, stay flexible, and have fun with the process. Happy meal planning!

3

Planning Strategies

Meal planning is a crucial part of eating healthy and staying organized in the kitchen. Planning strategies can range from weekly meal planning to batch cooking and freezer meals. In this chapter, we will discuss three effective planning strategies to help you save time and money in the kitchen.

Weekly Meal Planning

Weekly meal planning is a popular strategy that involves planning out all of your meals for the upcoming week. This can be done on a Sunday or whichever day is most convenient for you. The idea behind weekly meal planning is to have a plan in place for every meal, so you don't have to stress about what to make each day.

To start weekly meal planning, create a list of all the meals you will eat for the week. This can include breakfast, lunch, dinner, and snacks. Once you have a list of meals, create a shopping list of all the ingredients you will need. Be sure to check your pantry and fridge to see what ingredients you already have on hand, so you don't end up buying unnecessary items.

Once you have your shopping list, head to the grocery store and buy everything you need for the week. Once you are home, you can start preparing meals as needed. Many people find it helpful to do some meal prep on the weekend, such as chopping vegetables or cooking grains, to make meal preparation during the week faster and more efficient.

The benefits of weekly meal planning include saving time and money by avoiding unnecessary trips to the grocery store, reducing food waste by using ingredients before they spoil, and eating healthier by planning balanced meals in advance.

Batch Cooking

Batch cooking is another planning strategy that involves cooking a large amount of food at once and then portioning it out for future meals. This can be a great way to save time and money while still enjoying delicious, healthy meals throughout the week.

To start batch cooking, choose a recipe that can be easily scaled up to make a large amount of food. Good options include stews, soups, casseroles, and chili. Once you have your recipe, gather all the ingredients and start cooking. You can make a large pot of soup or chili, for example, and then portion it out into individual containers for future meals.

Batch cooking has many benefits, including saving time by reducing the need for daily meal preparation, saving money by buying ingredients in bulk, and reducing food waste by using up ingredients before they spoil.

Freezer Meals

Freezer meals are another planning strategy that involves preparing meals in advance and freezing them for future use. This can be a great option for busy families or individuals who don't have a lot of time to spend in the kitchen.

To start making freezer meals, choose recipes that freeze well, such as casseroles, soups, and stews. Once you have your recipes, gather all the ingredients and start cooking. Once the meals are cooked, portion them out into individual containers or freezer bags and label them with the date and contents.

The benefits of freezer meals include saving time by having pre-made meals on hand, saving money by buying ingredients in bulk, and reducing food waste by using up ingredients before they spoil.

Tips for Successful Planning Strategies

Here are some tips for successful meal planning strategies:

1. **Plan ahead:** The key to successful meal planning is to plan ahead. Whether you are doing weekly meal planning, batch

cooking, or freezer meals, it's important to have a plan in place before you start cooking.

2. **Make a shopping list:** Always make a shopping list before you head to the grocery store. This will help you stay organized and avoid buying unnecessary items.

3. **Use what you have:** Check your pantry and fridge before you go grocery shopping. This will help you use up ingredients that you already have on hand and reduce food waste.

4. **Keep it simple**: Don't try to make elaborate meals every day. Instead, focus on simple, healthy meals that can be prepared quickly and easily.

5. **Stay flexible:** Remember to stay flexible and be willing to adjust your meal plan as needed. Life can be unpredictable, so it's important to be adaptable.

6. **Get the whole family involved:** Meal planning can be a fun and educational activity for the whole family. Get everyone involved in choosing recipes and helping with meal prep.

7. **Try new recipes:** Don't be afraid to try new recipes and ingredients. This can help you stay motivated and interested in meal planning.

8. **Keep track of your progress:** Keep track of your progress by recording your meals, grocery expenses, and progress towards your goals. This can help you stay motivated and see the positive changes that meal planning can bring to your life.

By following these tips and strategies, you can make meal planning a successful and enjoyable part of your routine. Whether you are doing weekly meal planning, batch cooking, or freezer meals, remember to stay organized, stay flexible, and have fun with the process. Happy meal planning!

4

Building a Shopping List

Building a shopping list is an essential part of meal planning. A well-planned shopping list can help you save time and money, reduce food waste, and ensure that you have all the ingredients you need to make healthy, satisfying meals. In this chapter, we will discuss three strategies for building a successful shopping list: creating a master list of pantry staples, planning for weekly shopping trips, and utilizing sales and coupons.

Creating a Master List of Pantry Staples

Creating a master list of pantry staples is a great way to ensure that you always have the essential ingredients on hand to make meals. This list should include items that you use frequently and can be stored for a long time, such as canned goods, grains, and spices.

To create your master list, start by going through your pantry and taking note of the items that you use frequently. Some examples might include canned tomatoes, beans, rice, pasta, and flour. Once you have a list of pantry staples, keep it in a convenient place, such as on the fridge or in your meal planning notebook.

When you are planning your meals for the week, refer to your master list and cross off any items that you already have on hand. This will help you avoid buying unnecessary items and ensure that you always have the essentials on hand.

Planning for Weekly Shopping Trips

Planning for weekly shopping trips is another key strategy for building a successful shopping list. By planning ahead, you can ensure that you have all the ingredients you need for the week ahead, and avoid last-minute trips to the grocery store.

To plan for your weekly shopping trips, start by creating a list of all the meals you plan to make for the week. Once you have your list of meals, create a shopping list of all the ingredients you will need. Be sure to check your pantry and fridge for any items you already have on hand, so you don't end up buying duplicates.

When planning for your weekly shopping trip, consider the time of day and day of the week. Grocery stores tend to be less crowded early in the morning and late at night, so if you can, plan your trip for these times. You may also want to avoid going to the grocery store on weekends, when it tends to be more crowded.

Utilizing Sales and Coupons

Utilizing sales and coupons can be a great way to save money on your grocery bill. Many grocery stores offer weekly sales and promotions, as well as coupons that can be used to save money on specific items.

To take advantage of sales and coupons, start by reviewing the weekly sales flyers for your local grocery stores. Look for items that are on sale that you can incorporate into your meal plan for the week. You can also search for coupons online or in your local newspaper.

When using coupons, be sure to check the expiration date and any restrictions or limitations. Some coupons may be limited to a certain number of items, or may only be valid on certain days of the week.

Tips for Building a Successful Shopping List

Here are some tips for building a successful shopping list:

Plan ahead: The key to building a successful shopping list is to plan ahead. Take the time to plan your meals for the week and create a shopping list of all the ingredients you will need.

Use a shopping list app: Consider using a shopping list app, such as AnyList or Out of Milk, to keep track of your shopping list. These apps can be synced with multiple devices, so everyone in your household can add items to the list.

Stick to your list: When you are at the grocery store, stick to your list as much as possible. Avoid impulse purchases and stick to your meal plan for the week.

Shop the perimeter: When you are at the grocery store, focus on shopping the perimeter of the store, which is where the fresh produce, meat, and dairy products are located. This will help you avoid the processed and packaged foods in the center aisles.

Buy in bulk: Buying in bulk can be a cost-effective way to save money on groceries. Look for bulk bins for items such as grains, nuts, and dried fruits.

Check unit prices: When comparing prices, be sure to check the unit price of the item. This will help you determine which item is the best value.

Bring your own bags: Bringing your own reusable bags to the grocery store can help you save money and reduce waste.

By utilizing sales and coupons and building a successful shopping list, you can save money on groceries and ensure that you have everything you need to make healthy, budget-friendly meals. Remember to plan ahead, stick to your list, and focus on buying whole, nutritious foods. Happy shopping!

5

Preparing and Storing Meals

Preparing and storing meals is an important aspect of meal planning. By preparing meals in advance, you can save time and ensure that you always have healthy, satisfying meals on hand. Proper storage is also crucial for ensuring that your meals stay fresh and safe to eat. In this chapter, we will discuss meal prepping techniques, proper storage methods, and reheating and serving suggestions.

Meal Prepping Techniques

Meal prepping involves preparing ingredients or entire meals in advance to make mealtime easier and more efficient. There are several meal prepping techniques to choose from, depending on your preferences and needs.

One popular meal prepping technique is to prepare a large batch of a recipe, such as a soup, stew, or chili, and then portion it out into individual containers for future meals. This is a great option for busy individuals or families who don't have a lot of time to spend in the kitchen.

Another meal prepping technique is to prepare ingredients in advance, such as chopping vegetables or cooking grains. This can save time during meal preparation, as the ingredients are already prepped and ready to go.

Proper Storage Methods

Proper storage is crucial for ensuring that your meals stay fresh and safe to eat. Here are some tips for proper storage:

Use airtight containers: Use airtight containers, such as glass jars or plastic containers with tight-fitting lids, to store your meals. This will help keep your food fresh and prevent it from absorbing odors from other foods in the fridge.

Label and date containers: Label each container with the name of the dish and the date it was prepared. This will help you keep track of what's in your fridge and ensure that you eat meals before they spoil.

Store in the fridge or freezer: Store meals in the fridge for up to three to four days or in the freezer for up to three months.

Use freezer-safe containers: If you are storing meals in the freezer, be sure to use freezer-safe containers. Glass jars can break when frozen, so it's best to use plastic containers or freezer bags.

Reheating and Serving Suggestions

When it comes to reheating and serving meals, there are several options to choose from. Here are some suggestions:

Microwave: If you are short on time, the microwave is a quick and easy way to reheat meals. Simply place the meal in a microwave-safe container and heat for one to two minutes, or until heated through.

Oven: For meals that need to be crispy or browned, the oven is a good option. Place the meal in an oven-safe container and heat at 350°F for 10 to 15 minutes, or until heated through.

Stovetop: For meals that need to be heated slowly or stirred, such as soups or stews, the stovetop is a good option. Place the meal in a pot and heat over low to medium heat until heated through.

Garnishes and toppings: Adding garnishes and toppings to your meals can make them more flavorful and interesting. Consider adding fresh herbs, chopped nuts, or a dollop of yogurt or sour cream to your meals.

Serve with sides: Consider serving your meals with a side salad or roasted vegetables to make them more balanced and satisfying.

Tips for Successful Meal Preparation and Storage

Here are some tips for successful meal preparation and storage:

Choose recipes that freeze well: When choosing recipes to prepare in advance, consider choosing ones that freeze well, such as soups, stews, and casseroles.

Invest in high-quality storage containers: Investing in high-quality storage containers can make a big difference in the freshness and quality of your meals. Look for containers that are freezer-safe and have tight-fitting lids to prevent freezer burn.

Label and date your meals: Be sure to label and date your meals before storing them in the fridge or freezer. This will help you keep track of what you have on hand and ensure that you use up meals before they go bad.

Store meals in portion sizes: When storing meals, consider storing them in portion sizes that are appropriate for your needs. This will help you avoid wasting food and ensure that you have the right amount of food on hand.

Thaw meals safely: When thawing frozen meals, be sure to thaw them safely in the fridge or microwave. Avoid leaving meals out on the counter to thaw, as this can lead to the growth of harmful bacteria.

By following these tips for reheating and serving meals, as well as for meal preparation and storage, you can ensure that your meals are safe, fresh, and flavorful. Remember to use high-quality storage containers, label and date your meals, and thaw meals safely to avoid foodborne illness. Happy meal prepping!

6

Recipe Ideas

Meal planning can be a challenge, especially when you are trying to balance health, budget, and taste. In this chapter, we will provide some recipe ideas that are healthy, budget-friendly, and easy to prepare. We will also provide meal ideas for breakfast, lunch, and dinner, as well as vegetarian and vegan options.

Healthy and Budget-Friendly Recipes

Eating healthy on a budget can be a challenge, but there are many recipes that are both nutritious and affordable. Here are some healthy and budget-friendly recipe ideas:

1. **One-pot meals:** One-pot meals, such as soups, stews, and chili, are a great option for a healthy and budget-friendly meal. They can be made in large batches, which can save you time and money in the long run.
2. **Veggie stir-fry:** Stir-fries are another healthy and budget-friendly option. You can use a variety of vegetables, such

as broccoli, bell peppers, and carrots, and add in some tofu or chicken for protein.

3. **Lentil soup:** Lentils are a great source of protein and fiber, and lentil soup is a simple and delicious way to incorporate them into your meals. Add in some vegetables, such as carrots and celery, and spices, such as cumin and coriander, for a flavorful and satisfying soup.

4. **Baked sweet potatoes:** Sweet potatoes are a nutrient-dense and affordable option for a meal. You can bake them in the oven and top them with black beans, avocado, and salsa for a delicious and filling meal.

Meal Ideas for Breakfast, Lunch, and Dinner

Here are some meal ideas for breakfast, lunch, and dinner:

1. **Breakfast:** For a quick and easy breakfast, consider making overnight oats. Simply mix together oats, almond milk, chia seeds, and your favorite toppings, such as fruit and nuts, and let it sit in the fridge overnight.

2. **Lunch:** For a healthy and satisfying lunch, consider making a salad with mixed greens, grilled chicken, roasted vegetables, and a simple vinaigrette.

3. **Dinner:** For a hearty and comforting dinner, consider making a vegetable lasagna with layers of roasted vegetables, whole wheat noodles, and tomato sauce.

Vegetarian and Vegan Options

If you are vegetarian or vegan, there are many options available for healthy and delicious meals. Here are some vegetarian and vegan recipe ideas:

1. **Vegan chili:** Vegan chili is a flavorful and protein-packed option for a meal. You can use a variety of vegetables, such as sweet potatoes and bell peppers, and add in some black beans and spices, such as chili powder and cumin.
2. **Quinoa and black bean salad:** Quinoa is a great source of protein and fiber, and can be used in a variety of recipes. Consider making a quinoa and black bean salad with cherry tomatoes, avocado, and cilantro for a fresh and flavorful meal.
3. **Lentil shepherd's pie:** Lentils can be used as a meat substitute in many recipes, and lentil shepherd's pie is a delicious and comforting option. Simply layer cooked lentils with mashed potatoes and bake in the oven for a hearty and satisfying meal.

Tips for Successful Meal Planning and Recipe Ideas

Here are some tips for successful meal planning and recipe ideas:

1. **Keep it simple:** When planning your meals, keep it simple. Choose recipes that use simple ingredients and are easy to prepare.
2. **Use seasonal produce:** Using seasonal produce can save

you money and ensure that you are getting the freshest ingredients possible.

Make a list of go-to recipes: Keep a list of your favorite recipes that are healthy, easy to make, and budget-friendly. This will make meal planning easier in the long run, as you will have a variety of recipes to choose from.

Experiment with new ingredients: Don't be afraid to experiment with new ingredients and flavors. This can help you discover new favorite recipes and keep your meals interesting.

Prep in advance: Take advantage of your free time to prepare ingredients in advance, such as washing and chopping vegetables or cooking grains. This can help you save time during the week when you are busy.

Involve the whole family: Get the whole family involved in meal planning and preparation. This can be a fun and educational activity for everyone, and can help encourage healthy eating habits.

By following these tips and trying out vegetarian and vegan recipe ideas, you can make meal planning a successful and enjoyable part of your routine. Remember to keep it simple, use seasonal produce, experiment with new ingredients, prep in advance, and involve the whole family. Happy meal planning!

7

Tips for Success

Meal planning can be a great way to save time, money, and stress in the kitchen. However, it can also be challenging to make it a habit and overcome common obstacles. In this chapter, we will discuss tips for making meal planning a habit, troubleshooting common challenges, and celebrating your successes.

Making Meal Planning a Habit

Making meal planning a habit takes time and effort, but the benefits are worth it. Here are some tips for making meal planning a habit:

Schedule a dedicated meal planning time: Set aside a specific time each week to plan your meals. This will help you stay consistent and make it a regular part of your routine.

Start small: If meal planning is new to you, start small. Plan a few meals for the week and gradually work your way up to planning more.

Involve your family: If you live with others, involve them in the meal planning process. This can help you get input on what meals they would like to eat and make the process more enjoyable.

Keep it flexible: Meal planning doesn't have to be rigid. Leave some room for spontaneity and flexibility, such as planning for a takeout night or leftovers.

Troubleshooting Common Challenges

Meal planning can come with its own set of challenges. Here are some common challenges and how to overcome them:

Lack of time: If you are short on time, consider meal prepping on the weekends or using quick and easy recipes.

Limited kitchen space: If you have limited kitchen space, focus on meals that require minimal equipment and prep time.

Picky eaters: If you have picky eaters in your household, involve them in the meal planning process and try to incorporate their preferences into the meals.

Limited budget: If you are on a limited budget, focus on meals that use affordable ingredients and plan your meals around sales and coupons.

Celebrating Successes

Celebrating your successes can help you stay motivated and make meal planning a more enjoyable process. Here are some ways to celebrate your successes:

Share your meals with others: Share your meals with friends or family members and get their feedback. This can help you feel proud of your accomplishments and get inspiration for future meals.

Take pictures: Take pictures of your meals and share them on social media. This can help you get feedback and encouragement from others.

Treat yourself: Treat yourself to a special meal or snack after successfully completing a week of meal planning. This can help you feel motivated to continue the habit.

Tips for Success

Here are some additional tips for success:

Stay organized: Keep your meal planning notebook or app organized and up-to-date. This will help you stay on track and avoid last-minute trips to the grocery store.

Don't be too hard on yourself: Remember that meal planning is a process, and it's okay to make mistakes or have a week where things don't go as planned. Don't be too hard on yourself and use it as a learning experience.

Have fun with it: Meal planning can be a fun and creative process. Experiment with new recipes and ingredients and enjoy the process.

Make it a habit: The more you practice meal planning, the easier it will become. Make it a regular part of your routine and before you know it, it will become a habit.

Meal planning can be a great way to save time, money, and stress in the kitchen. By following these tips for success and staying organized, you can make meal planning a habit and enjoy the benefits of healthy, budget-friendly meals that can be prepared in advance. Remember to stay flexible, celebrate your successes, and have fun with them.

8

Final Thoughts

Meal planning is a powerful tool for taking control of your health and budget. It can help you save time, reduce stress, and make healthier choices. In this chapter, we will recap the benefits of meal planning and provide encouragement to start meal planning today.

Recap of Benefits

Here is a recap of the benefits of meal planning:

Saves time: Meal planning can save you time in the kitchen by reducing the time you spend grocery shopping and preparing meals.

Saves money: Meal planning can save you money by reducing food waste, helping you take advantage of sales and coupons, and encouraging you to eat out less.

Improves health: Meal planning can improve your health by encouraging you to make healthier choices and control portion sizes.

Reduces stress: Meal planning can reduce stress by taking the guesswork out of mealtime and reducing the need for last-minute trips to the grocery store or fast food restaurants.

Encouragement to Start Meal Planning

If you haven't started meal planning yet, now is the time to start. Here are some tips to get started:

Choose a day and time to plan: Choose a day and time each week to plan your meals. This will help you stay consistent and make it a regular part of your routine.

Gather recipe ideas: Gather recipe ideas from cookbooks, websites, and social media. Look for healthy and budget-friendly recipes that appeal to your tastes.

Make a grocery list: Make a grocery list based on the meals you have planned for the week. Check your pantry and fridge to see what you already have on hand.

Meal prep in advance: Consider meal prepping in advance by cooking ingredients, such as grains or roasted vegetables, or preparing entire meals in advance.

Stay flexible: Remember to stay flexible and make adjustments as needed. Don't be afraid to switch up meals or adjust portion sizes based on your appetite.

Meal planning is a valuable tool for taking control of your health and budget. By following the tips and strategies outlined in this guide, you can start meal planning today and enjoy the benefits of healthy, budget-friendly meals that can be prepared in advance. Remember to stay organized, stay flexible, and have fun with the process. Happy meal planning!

9

Glossary

Meal planning can involve many terms and concepts that may be unfamiliar to some. In this chapter, we will provide a glossary of common meal planning terms to help you better understand the process.

1. **Meal planning:** The process of planning out meals in advance, typically for a week or longer.
2. **Batch cooking:** The practice of cooking large batches of food, such as soups or casseroles, and then dividing them into portions for future meals.
3. **Freezer meals:** Meals that are prepared in advance and frozen for later use.
4. **Meal prep:** The process of preparing ingredients or entire meals in advance to make mealtime easier and more efficient.
5. **Pantry staples:** Basic ingredients that are typically kept on hand in the pantry, such as canned goods, grains, and spices.
6. **Sales and coupons:** Discounts and promotions offered by

grocery stores to encourage purchases.

7. **Airtight containers:** Containers with tight-fitting lids that prevent air from entering, helping to keep food fresh.

8. **Reheating:** The process of heating up previously cooked food.

9. **Storing:** The process of keeping food in a safe and appropriate place, such as the fridge or freezer.

10. **Meal plan template:** A document or tool used to plan out meals for the week or month.

11. **Nutritional information:** Information about the nutritional value of a particular food or meal, such as calories, fat content, and protein content.

12. **Vegetarian:** A person who does not eat meat, including fish and poultry.

13. **Vegan:** A person who does not consume any animal products, including meat, dairy, and eggs.

14. **Budget-friendly:** A term used to describe meals or ingredients that are affordable and fit within a specific budget.

15. **Portion control:** The practice of controlling the amount of food consumed at each meal to ensure proper nutrition and prevent overeating.

16. **Recipe modification:** The process of making changes to a recipe, such as reducing fat or adding more vegetables.

17. **Shopping list:** A list of items needed for meal preparation and other household needs.

18. **Meal rotation:** The practice of rotating meals to prevent boredom and ensure a variety of nutrients.

19. **Food waste:** The amount of food that is discarded or thrown away.

20. **Leftovers:** Food that is leftover from a previous meal and can be eaten later.

By familiarizing yourself with these common meal planning terms, you can better understand the process and make informed decisions about your meal planning strategies.

10

Additional Resources

In addition to the information provided in this guide, there are many resources available to help you with your meal planning journey. In this chapter, we will provide a list of additional resources to help you plan healthy, budget-friendly meals that can be prepared in advance.

Cookbooks: There are many cookbooks available that focus on healthy, budget-friendly meals and meal planning strategies. Some popular options include "The Budget-Friendly Fresh and Local Diabetes Cookbook" by Charles Mattocks and "The Healthy Meal Prep Cookbook" by Toby Amidor.

Meal planning apps: There are several apps available that can help you with meal planning, grocery shopping, and tracking your food intake. Some popular options include Mealime, Plan to Eat, and Meal Planner Pro.

Online resources: There are many websites and blogs that offer meal planning tips, recipes, and grocery shopping strategies.

Some popular options include Budget Bytes, Skinnytaste, and Eating Well.

Meal delivery services: If you are short on time or prefer not to cook, meal delivery services can be a convenient option. Services such as HelloFresh, Blue Apron, and Freshly deliver pre-portioned ingredients and recipes directly to your doorstep.

Local resources: Check with your local grocery store or community center for resources on healthy eating and meal planning. Some stores offer cooking classes or meal planning workshops, and community centers may offer resources such as community gardens or nutrition education programs.

Registered Dietitian Nutritionists (RDNs): RDNs can provide personalized meal planning and nutrition advice based on your individual needs and goals. To find a registered dietitian in your area, visit the Academy of Nutrition and Dietetics website.

By utilizing these additional resources, you can gain more knowledge and support to make meal planning a successful and enjoyable part of your routine.

11

Bonus: Templates

Weekly Meal Planning Template

Monday:
  Breakfast:
  Lunch:
  Dinner:

Tuesday:
  Breakfast:
  Lunch:
  Dinner:

Wednesday:
  Breakfast:
  Lunch:
  Dinner:

Thursday:

Breakfast:
Lunch:
Dinner:

Friday:
Breakfast:
Lunch:
Dinner:

Saturday:
Breakfast:
Lunch:
Dinner:

Sunday:
Breakfast:
Lunch:
Dinner:

Daily Meal Planning Template

Breakfast:
Snack:
Lunch:
Snack:
Dinner:
Snack:

Batch Cooking Meal Planning Template

Monday:
  Lunch: Leftover Chili
  Dinner: Slow Cooker Chicken and Vegetables

Tuesday:
  Lunch: Slow Cooker Chicken and Vegetables
  Dinner: Leftover Chili

Wednesday:
  Lunch: Slow Cooker Chicken and Vegetables
  Dinner: Chicken Stir-Fry

Thursday:
  Lunch: Chicken Stir-Fry
  Dinner: Leftover Chili

Friday:
  Lunch: Chicken Stir-Fry
  Dinner: Slow Cooker Beef Stew

Saturday:
  Lunch: Slow Cooker Beef Stew
  Dinner: Chicken Stir-Fry

Sunday:
  Lunch: Slow Cooker Beef Stew
  Dinner: Leftover Chili

These meal planning templates can help you stay organized

and ensure that you are meeting your dietary needs and budget limits. Feel free to customize them to fit your specific needs and preferences. Happy meal planning!

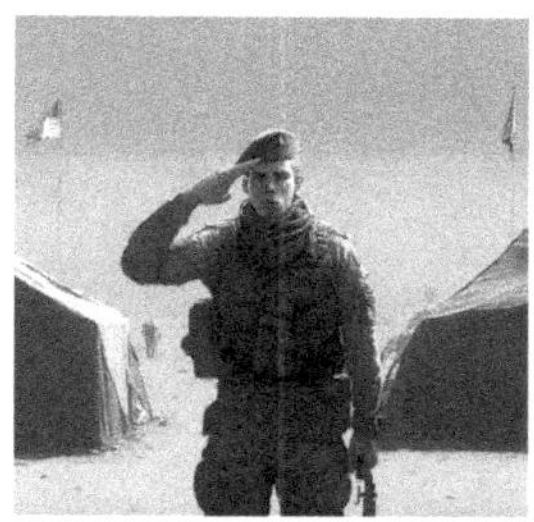

About the Author

Avery Wright is an enigmatic figure who is an author in the fields of AI, Technology, and the Arts. A combat veteran of the US Army, Avery has almost two decades of experience in the IT industry, which has given them a unique perspective on the intersection of technology and society.

As an author, Avery has published a range of books on topics such as the future of AI, the role of drones in modern warfare, and the medicinal properties of mushrooms. Their writing often explores the cutting-edge of technology and how it is changing the world around us. Avery's work is notable for its depth and insight, as well as its ability to make complex topics accessible to a broad audience.

Away from the world of writing, Avery is a private individual who values their privacy. Despite this, they remain a voice in the tech industry and beyond. Whether sharing their thoughts on the latest developments in AI or commenting on the state of the world, Avery's perspective is always worth listening to.

You can connect with me on:

- https://sirexodia.wixsite.com/avery-wright
- https://twitter.com/AveryWrightAI
- https://www.facebook.com/profile.php?id=100089987171726
- https://www.amazon.com/author/averywrightai

Subscribe to my newsletter:

- https://sirexodia.wixsite.com/avery-wright

Also by Avery Wright

Also by Avery Wright

"Mastering Midjourney AI: The Beginner's Handbook"

"Chat GPT: A Digital Journey Begins"

"AI and the Art of Binary"

"Mycological Marvels: Exploring the Art of AI-Created Mushrooms"

"AI in Healthcare: How Artificial Intelligence is Transforming Medicine"

"Transformative Art:: A Journey with Artificial Intelligence"

"From Predator to Phantom: A Glimpse At Drones"

"AI and the Future of Humanity"

"The Tao of Inner Peace"

"Taoism Unleashed: Advanced Concepts for Deepening Your Practice"

"The Knife's Edge:: A View on the Ultra Rich and their Motivations"

"Defending the Skies: The Rise of Unidentified Aerial Phenomena and the Battle for Airspace Dominance"

"Mastering the Board: The Power of Pawns in Chess"

"The Brain in the Machine: Understanding the Inner Workings of Artificial Intelligence"

"Healing with Fungi: The Science of Medicinal Mushrooms"

"Chat GPT: ChatGPT Explores the World: Conversations Across Cultures"

"Chat GPT: Unleashing ChatGPT's Power: Navigating the Digital Realm"

Avery Wright's work spans a range of topics, from the cutting-edge of AI and technology to the ancient practice of Taoism and the art of chess. Their books are notable for their depth, insight, and ability to make complex topics accessible to a broad audience. With almost two decades of experience in the IT field and a background as a combat veteran, Avery brings a unique perspective to their writing that is both informative and thought-provoking. Whether you are interested in exploring the frontiers of technology or deepening your understanding of the human experience, Avery's books are a must-read.

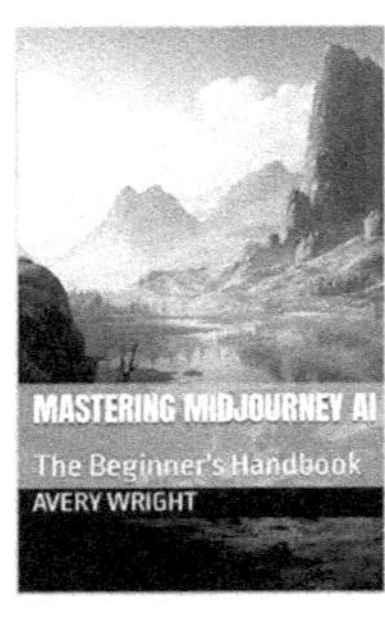

Mastering Midjourney AI - The Beginner's Handbook

Mastering Midjourney AI: The Beginner's Handbook is a comprehensive guide for beginners looking to learn about the Midjourney AI platform and how to use it for image generation. The book covers a range of topics, including understanding Midjourney AI's parameters and settings, using URLs for image inspiration, adjusting image quality, and more.

https://www.amazon.com/dp/B0BV8PGDXT

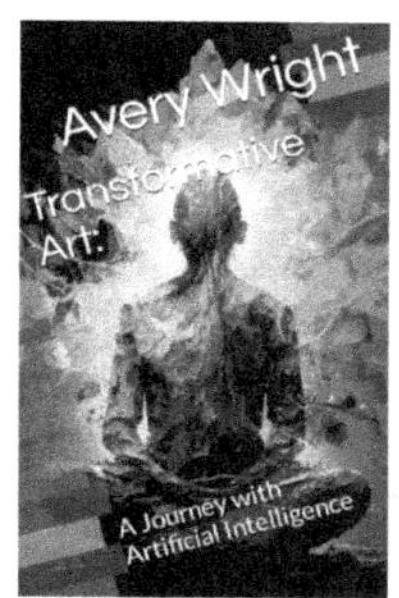

Transformative Art – A Journey with Artificial Intelligence

Transformative Art: A Journey with AI is a visually stunning and thought-provoking book that explores the intersection of artificial intelligence and the world of art. The book features breathtaking images of futuristic cities, technology, vehicles, robots, flying ships, conceptual art, abstract art, and unique pieces, all within the context of transformative art. Each chapter begins with a powerful quote that sets the tone for a deep dive into the themes of perception, change, reflection, risk-taking, emotional connection, the journey within, and the universal language of art. The book is written by Avery Wright, a talented author with a passion for exploring the ways in which technology is changing our lives and our world. This book is a must-read for anyone interested in the intersection of art, technology, and the human experience. https://www.amazon.com/dp/B0BTWNYLJD

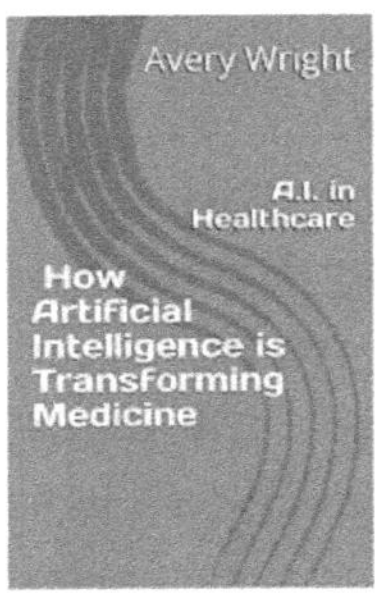

AI in Healthcare: How Artificial Intelligence is Transforming Medicine

Discover the groundbreaking impact of AI in healthcare. From personalized medicine to revolutionizing the healthcare workforce, AI is changing the game. Get a deeper understanding of its current and future applications and the ethical, legal, and social implications in "AI in Healthcare: How Artificial Intelligence is Transforming Medicine." Get your copy now on Amazon!

https://www.amazon.com/dp/B0BTBZDVBY

AI and the Art of Binary

"Binary and AI: The Art of Computer Science" delves into the world of binary and its applications in artificial intelligence. The book starts with an explanation of binary and its relationship with computer science, followed by an in-depth exploration of the different applications of binary in AI, including machine learning, natural language processing, computer vision, and robotics. The book also covers the coding aspect of binary for AI and provides the reader with best practices and tools used for coding.

https://www.amazon.com/dp/B0BV5RK9ZG

Remembering a Different Past: The Fascinating World of Mandela Effects

Remembering a Different Past: The Fascinating World of Mandela Effects is a captivating exploration of the phenomenon known as the Mandela Effect. This book delves into the world of memory, perception, and reality, challenging our understanding of the nature of truth and knowledge. Through a mixture of personal experiences, research, and scientific exploration, this book will leave you questioning the reliability of your own memories and perceptions.